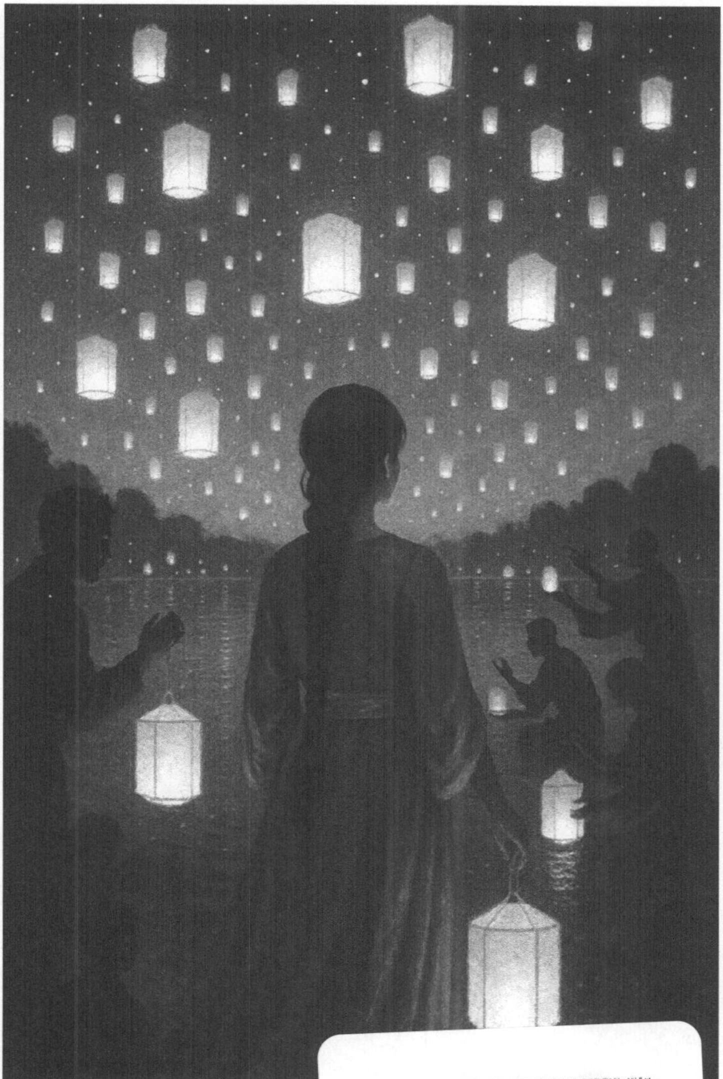

First Published by Ink Gladiators Press®

Translations Of Hope

Editor-in-Chief: Reena Doss

First Edition
ISBN 13: 978-93-49117-40-2

Bottled Sounds For You - Lantern 4

Credits:
Book Design by Leonie Belle Hawk
Sanskrit & Swedish Translations: Edited and Proofed
by Justin Adam Wolf and Aelius Arche

Ink Gladiators Press®
Publishing and promoting warriors on life's battlefield
Founded in 2019 | Bangalore, India
www.inkgladiatorspress.com

To my beloved Weaver,

Thank you for sharing your love of sound with us
so that we could discover how to interpret them in our way;
this is my thankful note to you for opening my heart
to feel the sound of music woven into the works of others

To my future family,

you are the ones I imagine before me
when I write a book, create art, share reflections or feel music;
may we each find joy in our gifted voices of expression,
whether as listeners, artists, writers, musicians, singers,
lyricists, creatives or all of them

To my dear Gardeners,

You are so many that I find it hard to name all
but you each planted seeds in my life that I found on this path;
may you never stop sharing your passion for instruments

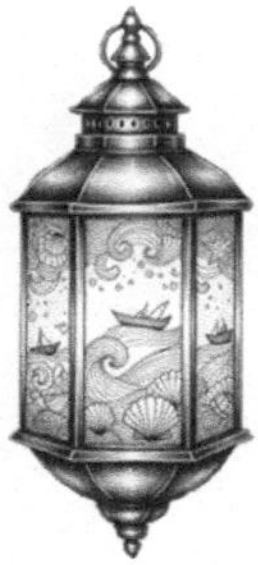

This book is a lantern of

Bottled Sounds For You

Love Adores
Never-ending Tales:
Eagerly Ready, News Sails

The main content is written in English, with their Sanskrit and Swedish translations added after each piece.
Here is the link to listen while you read this booklet:
https://tinyurl.com/bottledsounds

Bottled Sounds For You

Because Mental Health Matters

I stopped numbering my pages because my story is still being written.

Besides, I do like its symbol a lot—a sleeping 8.

I'll find you in the dark because I'm the girl

who loves to stay *lost* amongst the midnight stars

caught up with moonbeams *in a lantern*

trying to find my way back *home*

LANTERNS

The pleasure of watching light move across the night sky against its deep purples, blues and greys is an incredible sight to behold.

Though I have never seen it in person myself except on TV, reels or videos, I would imagine that it mimics the feeling of a thousand golden suns glimmering brighter than the stars behind them. I would imagine that it would capture the feeling of remembering that we are each important because no matter how small or big we are light travels faster than sound. I would imagine it would make anyone who sees them smile, open their hearts as hope flutters like birdsong near their door, and the taste of something indescribably good wraps them warmly.

Lanterns are necessary because igniting hope is the best cure in support of mental health awareness. Many live in darkness, in a state of feeling disillusioned by those they put their faith in and have forgotten how to see their own hearts through eyes that love, but a lantern is meant for just this purpose—to relight someone's candle with kindness, to hold a hand steadily in their shadows, and to listen gently to the broken pieces in others speaking. Sometimes, the truth is simple.

That delicate point between human nature and the desire to do what is good is where we will meet the Author of Love. Love can only be known from the One who created us and even when people (who follow God) make us feel like He isn't real or there for us, one of the best ways to reconnect with Him directly is to love with all your heart—and to balance it with healthy discernment, boundaries and truth in situations where your broken parts might want to do, feel or say the exact opposite. *E.g.: Jesus Christ*

It is my joy to let go of this lantern—as all lanterns must be—for others to find because I want to share something beautiful that I gained and that is mine to offer: You are deeply loved by Heavenly Hands that have constructed, created and command time, space, and distance.

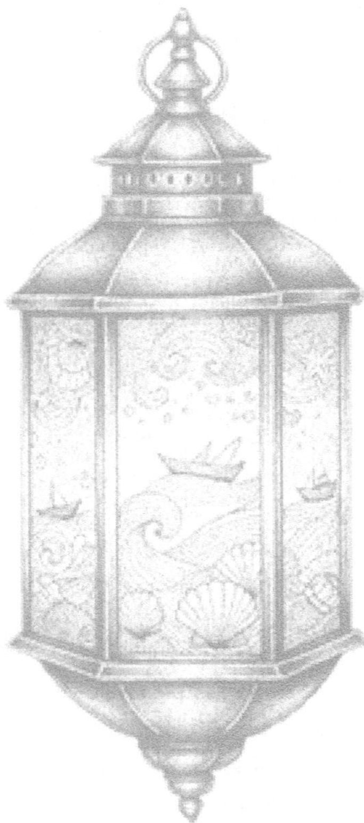

∞

Guitar

The gravitational fire of passion burns in the strumming of a guitarist. Ever heard the way their fingers crash into the strings? There is a ravishing that occurs between the instrument and the music of the heart who plays it. And when you relate to the emotions they unveil in the depths of the nuances they evoke; it is like touching the soul of someone who feels everything that you do.

Let Me Down Slowly by Joni Laakkonen

गिटारः

गिटारवादकस्य तारस्पन्दनेषु कामस्य गुरुत्वाकर्षणवत् अग्निः दहति। कदा तव श्रुतं यथा तेषां अङ्गुलीनां तारैः सङ्घर्षः? वाद्ययन्त्रस्य च तं वादनं कुर्वतः हृदयसङ्गीतस्य च मध्ये एकः मनोहरः मेलः जायते। यदा च त्वं तेषां सूक्ष्मतत्त्वेषु उद्घाटितानां भावनानां सहानुभूतिं कुर्वसि, तदा यथा त्वया यत् किञ्चित् अनुभूतम्, तत् सर्वं अनुभूतवान् कस्यचित् आत्मानं स्पृशसि इव।

जोनी लाक्कोनेन रचितं 'लेट् मी डाउन् स्लोली'

Gitarr

Den gravitationella elden av passion brinner i gitarristens strumming. Har du någonsin hört hur deras fingrar slår mot strängarna? Det uppstår en hänförande känsla mellan instrumentet och musiken i hjärtat hos den som spelar. Och när du relaterar till de känslor som de avslöjar i djupet av de nyanser de framkallar, är det som att röra vid själen hos någon som känner precis samma sak som du.

Let Me Down Slowly av Joni Laakkonen

Cello

It always feels like goosebumps arrive when the waves of this song are played on the strings by a cellist. How is it possible to capture in words the love it draws out of my soul? I suppose I can only write about it.

Eyes Closed by Vesislava

चेलो

यदा चेलोवादकः तन्तुषु अस्य गीतस्य तरङ्गान् वादयति, तदा रोमाञ्चः जायते इति सदा अनुभूयते। मम आत्मनात् यत् प्रेम सः आहरति, तत् कथं शब्दैः ग्रहीतुं शक्यते? मम मन्ये अहं केवलं तस्य विषये लिखितुं शक्नोमि।

आक्षिप्ताः नेत्राः, वेसिस्लावया

Cello

Det känns alltid som att jag får gåshud när cellisten spelar denna låt på strängarna. Hur är det möjligt att med ord beskriva den kärlek som den väcker i min själ? Jag antar att jag bara kan skriva om den.

Eyes Closed av Vesislava

Violin

I have no idea why my eyes fill with tears whenever any violinist plays this song. It's like the sadness in the depths of my soul gets to tenderly come to the surface of my heart and feel like it's okay to be free.

Never Enough by Mathew Castle

वायलिन

यदा कश्चित् वायलिनवादकः एतत् गीतं वादयति, तदा मम नेत्राणि अश्रुपूरितानि भवन्ति, किमर्थं इति मम न ज्ञायते। मम आत्मनः गभीरतायाम् विद्यमाना दुःखभावना मृदुतापूर्वकं हृदयपृष्ठे उदितुं शक्नोति इव, च स्वातन्त्र्यं स्वीकर्तुं उचितम् इति अनुभूयते।

नेवर् इन्फिच् (Never Enough) – मॅथ्यू क्यासल्

Violin

Jag har ingen aning om varför mina ögon fylls av tårar varje gång en violinist spelar denna låt. Det är som om sorgen i djupet av min själ kommer upp till ytan av mitt hjärta och känner att det är okej att vara fri.

Never Enough av Mathew Castle

Harp

There is a symphony between the layers of the strings that only a harpist can sense when they strum. It is like as if nostalgia and depth married each other and became hope.

Listen to Until I Found You by Arianna Worthen

वीणा

तन्तुपटलेषु एकः सङ्गीतसमन्वयः अस्ति, यः केवलं वीणावादकेन तन्तुस्पर्शे एव अनुभूतुं शक्यते। यथा भूतस्मृतिः गभीरता च परस्परं मिलित्वा आशां जाताः इव।

श्रृणु 'अन्टिल् आइ फाउण्ड यू' (एरियन्ना वर्थेन्)

Harpa

Det finns en symfoni mellan strängarnas lager som bara en harpist kan känna när de spelar. Det är som om nostalgi och djup gifte sig med varandra och blev till hopp.

Lyssna på Until I Found You av Arianna Worthen

∞

Piano

A soft hum in the lakes of my chest suddenly become swans of ethereal beauty, gliding in a ballet of their own design. I am not sure whether the wild in me acknowledges these sensations, but my fingers paint the music of their thoughts in words.

River Flows In You by Yiruma

पियानो

मम वक्षसि सरः इव मृदुं गुंजनं अकस्मात् दिव्यसौन्दर्ययुक्तैः हंसैः परिवर्तते, ये स्वयंकल्पितनृत्ये तरन्ति। मम अन्तर्निहितः वन्यभावः एतान् अनुभूतिम् अवगच्छति वा न, न जानामि; परन्तु मम अङ्गुलयः तेषां चिन्तनानां सङ्गीतं शब्दैः चित्रयन्ति।

'रिवर् फ्लोज् इन् यू' (यिरुमा)

Piano

Ett mjukt surrande i sjöarna i mitt bröst blir plötsligt svanar av eterisk skönhet, som glider i en balett av eget design. Jag är inte säker på om det vilda i mig erkänner dessa känslor, men mina fingrar målar musiken av deras tankar i ord.

River Flows In You av Yiruma

Irish Flute

I always feel as though I am under a hypnotised trance when I listen to the notes played by a flutist. It is like they have the most beautiful stories unravelling in the heart of their rhythm, but each one who listens will hear it differently based on the mood you are in. From start to finish, it is literally like they put a spell on you.

The Girl I'll Ne'er Forget by Matt Molloy

आयरिश् बांसुरी

यदा अहं बांसुरीवादकस्य स्वरान् शृणोमि, तदा मम मनः सम्मोहन-समाधौ स्थित इव अनुभवामि। यथा तेषां लये हृदि रमणीयाः कथाः प्रकटीभवन्ति, परन्तु श्रोता स्वभावेन भिन्नं श्रवणे अनुभवति। आरम्भात् समापनपर्यन्तम्, यथा ते तव मनसि मन्त्रं स्थापयन्ति इव।

मैट् मोलोय् रचितं 'या कन्या मया कदापि विस्मर्तुं न शक्यते'

Irländsk flöjt

Jag känner mig alltid som om jag är i trans när jag lyssnar på tonerna som spelas av en flöjtist. Det är som om de har de vackraste berättelserna som utvecklas i hjärtat av deras rytm, men varje lyssnare hör dem på olika sätt beroende på vilket humör man är på. Från början till slut är det bokstavligen som om de förtrollar en.

The Girl I'll Ne'er Forget av Matt Molloy

Santoor

There is a deep mystical quality in the emotional layers in the music created by a Santoorist. There is not just fine delicate feelings pulled at, there is also a sense of it being conducted to flow in a way that perplexes but also relieves you. You can feel the complexity as well as the raw sentiments moving in flow.

Zara Zara by Ninad Daithankar

संतूरः

संतूरवादकेन सृजिते सङ्गीते भावनात्मकस्तरेषु गभीरं रहस्यमयं गुणं अस्ति। न केवलं सूक्ष्माः कोमलभावनाः स्पृशन्ते, अपि तु तद् प्रवाहं निर्देशितं इति अनुभूयते, यः त्वां क्लिष्टं करोति परं च विमोचयति। त्वं जटिलतां च तथा कच्चभावनानां प्रवाहं च अनुभवितुं शक्नोषि।

झारा झारा – निनद् दैथंकरः

Santoor

Det finns en djup mystik i de emotionella lagren i musiken som skapas av en santoorist. Det är inte bara fina, delikata känslor som väcks, utan också en känsla av att den dirigeras för att flöda på ett sätt som förvirrar men också lindrar dig. Du kan känna komplexiteten och de råa känslorna som rör sig i flödet.

Zara Zara av Ninad Daithankar

Mandolin

When you listen to a Mandolinist, you just know they are speaking of a history that is still alive among them. They tell stories in the wilds of their soul without needing a map, facts or knowledge to be aware of something deep in their bones. To understand the music is almost not necessary because in its rhythm, one feels invited to be part of a known and unknown heritage of mystery, simply by feeling the warmth of hospitality in its symbolic tunes.

Come To The Sea by Music Of Italy

मण्डोलिन्

यदा मण्डोलिन्-वादकं शृणोषि, तदा त्वं अवगच्छसि यत् ते जीविते इतिहासे भाषन्ते। ते स्व-आत्मनः जङ्गलप्रदेशे कथाः कथयन्ति, न च मानचित्रं, न तथ्यानि, न ज्ञानं अपेक्ष्यते, यत् ते स्व-अस्थिषु गभीरं किञ्चित् अवगच्छन्ति। संगीतं अवगन्तुं प्रायः आवश्यकं नास्ति, यतः तस्य लये मानुषः केवलं तस्य प्रतीकात्मकस्वरेषु आतिथ्यस्य ऊष्णतां अनुभूत्वा परिचित-अपरिचित-रहस्यमय-परम्परायाः अङ्गत्वाय आमन्त्रितः इव अनुभवति।

इटालियायाः सङ्गीतेन 'समुद्रं आगच्छ'

Mandolin

När man lyssnar på en mandolinist vet man bara att de talar om en historia som fortfarande lever bland dem. De berättar historier i sin själs vildmark utan att behöva en karta, fakta eller kunskap för att vara medvetna om något djupt i sina ben. Det är nästan inte nödvändigt att förstå musiken, för i dess rytm känner man sig inbjuden att bli en del av ett känt och okänt arv av mystik, helt enkelt genom att känna värmen av gästfrihet i dess symboliska melodier.

Come To The Sea av Music Of Italy

Harmonica

There is something so pure, aesthetic and climatic in the sound a harmonist creates. It weeping in music of what and yet they make it sound like a story of love that was worth taking. Their music feels ocean born and cannot be explained unless I tell you in poetry that they are merfolk that have known heartbreak and ache of what can never be returned, only transformed.

Some Time When It Rains by Yang Han Fen

हार्मोनिका

हार्मोनिकावादकः यत् ध्वनिं सृजति तस्मिन् किञ्चित् विशुद्धं, सौन्दर्यपूर्णं च, उत्कर्षयुक्तं च अस्ति। सा ध्वनिः यथाशोकपूर्णं सङ्गीतरूपेण प्रवहति, तथापि तेन तं ध्वनिं रमणीयप्रेमकथायाः इव ध्वनयति, या स्वीक्रियते इति। तेषां सङ्गीतं समुद्रजातं इव अनुभूयते। यावत् अहं काव्येन न वदामि, तावत् तद् व्याख्यातुं न शक्यते। ते जलजनाः, ये हृदयभङ्गदुःखं च अनुभूतवन्तः, यत् कदापि प्रत्यागन्तुं न शक्यते, केवलं रूपान्तरितुं शक्यते।

याङ् हान् फेन् रचितम् 'कदाचित् यदा वर्षा भवति'

Harmonika

Det finns något så rent, estetiskt och stämningsfullt i den ljud som en harmonikaspelare skapar. Det gråter i musiken, men ändå får de det att låta som en kärlekshistoria som var värd att uppleva. Deras musik känns som om den är född i havet och kan inte förklaras annat än genom att jag berättar i poesi att de är sjöjungfrur som har upplevt hjärtesorg och smärtan av det som aldrig kan återvända, bara förvandlas.

Some Time When It Rains av Yang Han Fen

Lyre

The musical notes played by a lyrist carry me somewhere no one can follow. I suppose there is a reason why but when I listen I can reach intangible concepts and explain them fluently in poetry like why silver walks with the moon and threads itself into the edges that glow. It is fantasy storytelling in music form.

Echo by Lina Palera

लीरः

लीरवादकेन वादिताः सङ्गीतनादाः मां कुत्रापि वहन्ति यत्र अनुगन्तुं कश्चन न शक्नोति। कारणं किञ्चित् अस्ति इति मया मन्यते, परन्तु यदा अहं शृणोमि तदा अहं अमूर्तधारणाः प्राप्तुं शक्नोमि तथा तान् काव्येन सुबोधतया व्याख्यातुं शक्नोमि, यथा 'किमर्थं रजतं चन्द्रमया सह गच्छति तथा दीप्तिमान् सीमान् मध्ये स्वसूत्रं योजयति' इति। एतत् सङ्गीतरूपेण कल्पनाकथावाचनम् अस्ति।

प्रतिध्वनि – लीना पलेरा

Lyra

De toner som spelas av en lyraspelare för mig någonstans dit ingen kan följa efter. Jag antar att det finns en anledning till det, men när jag lyssnar kan jag nå immateriella begrepp och förklara dem flytande i poesi, som varför silver vandrar med månen och tränger sig in i kanterna som lyser. Det är fantasifullt berättande i musikform.

Echo av Lina Palera

Ukulele

The strings of this instrument make any notes strummed bring me a sense of melody that says "life will be okay". And sometimes, that's exactly what we need to remember. Because in that pause, I feel the chords of music reach over and tug my ears gently with no agenda except to just tune out with them.

Hey Jude by The O'Neill Brothers

उकुलेले

अस्य वाद्यस्य तन्तवः यदा कञ्चन स्वरं वादयन्ति, तदा मम मनसि रागाभासः जायते यः वदति - "जीवनं सम्यक् भविष्यति"। कदाचित् एतत् एव स्मरणं वयं कर्तुं इच्छामः। तस्मिन् विरामे अहं अनुभवामि यत् सङ्गीतस्वरसमूहः मम कर्णान् सौम्यतया आकरषति, केवलं तेषां सह विलीनं कर्तुं इति एव लक्ष्यं, अन्यत् किञ्चन नास्ति।

हे जूड़ – द ओ'नील् ब्रदर्स्

Ukulele

Strängarna på detta instrument gör att alla toner som spelas ger mig en känsla av melodi som säger "livet kommer att bli bra". Och ibland är det precis det vi behöver komma ihåg. För i den pausen känner jag att musikens ackord når fram och drar försiktigt i mina öron utan någon annan agenda än att bara stänga ute omvärlden med dem.

Hey Jude av The O'Neill Brothers

Mountain Dulcimer

Whenever I hear a dulcimerist, I can't help but think of midnight bonfires, times gone by and stories that feel like they will peel themselves out from the land, water or sky just because they want to sing with me. It is music that doesn't ask if it is welcome or not, it just chooses to make a home within your soul.

Danny Boy by Kevin Roth

पर्वत-डुल्सीमर्

यदा कदाचित् अहं डुल्सीमर्-वादकं श्रवामि, तदा मध्यरात्रिकाग्नयः, गताः कालाः, कथाश्च मम मनसि आगच्छन्ति, याः भूमिमात्रात् वा जलात् वा आकाशात् स्वयमेव निष्कास्यन्ते इव, केवलं मया सह गायितुं इच्छन्ति। एतत् संगीतम् स्वागतार्हम् वा न वा इति न पृच्छति, केवलं तव आत्मनि गृहं कर्तुम् इच्छति।

डैनी बॉय् – केविन् रोथ्

Mountain Dulcimer

När jag hör en dulcimerist kan jag inte låta bli att tänka på midnattseldar, svunna tider och berättelser som känns som om de kommer att lossna från marken, vattnet eller himlen bara för att de vill sjunga med mig. Det är musik som inte frågar om den är välkommen eller inte, den väljer bara att göra sig hemmastadd i din själ.

Danny Boy av Kevin Roth

Lute

In the classical strumming of its strings, I find myself contemplating life in generations before me. A lutenist has an uncanny ability to relax the mind and make me feel like I am walking in gardens of sunshine, valleys with trees of colour and dancing in castles rich with stories of adventures waiting to speak to me.

The Noble Man by Nigel North

ल्यूट्

तस्य तारवादनस्य शास्त्रीयस्पन्दने मया पूर्वपीढीनां जीवनम् अवलोक्य मननं भवति। ल्यूटवादकः मनः विश्रान्तिं दातुं अद्भुतां शक्तिं धारयति, यया मम अनुभूतिर्भवति यथा अहं सूर्यकिरणोद्यानेषु विचरन्, वर्णवृक्षयुक्तेषु उपत्यकासु च, कथासम्पन्नेषु दुर्गेषु नृत्यन् अस्मि।

दि नोबल् म्यान् – नाइजेल् नॉर्थ्

Luta

När jag hör det klassiska strummandet på strängarna finner jag mig själv fundera över livet i generationerna före mig. En lutspelare har en otrolig förmåga att få mig att slappna av och känna att jag vandrar i soliga trädgårdar, dalar med färgglada träd och dansar i slott fyllda med äventyrshistorier som väntar på att berättas för mig.

The Noble Man av Nigel North

Space For You

Bottled Sounds For You

Space For You

Reena Doss

Space For You

Acknowledgements

I am grateful

Music is a language I listen to. There is a peace in it that no unkindness can touch. I may not know the composers, or the history behind their inspirations or even how famous or unknown they probably are. If the music of your energy makes me feel—you can be a stranger and I will smile at you, unguarded...

This is the reason why I thank the Weaver for teaching me through the seeds planted by nature, humanity and the wild at different stages in my life about the beauty of sound when it is pure, creative and filled with the symphony of layered emotions felt, experienced and performed by the living.

Instruments for some reason find my voices: the spoken, written and silent ones. I name the chambers of my ink just like I give the people I meet the names of monuments or languages or connect them to the Wild Earth to describe the essence of who they are and how I feel and see them.

Guitars, violins, cellos and pianos play keys that make my mind take flight in the balance of all that my ink knows but I don't. But of all the instruments out there, I have always been drawn to the piano. There's something about the dance of fingers on black and white keys that makes think I'm playing with the waves and hearing its sounds of water, sunshine and falling rain.

I've never been formally taught so I don't always know the names of the keys or the correct way to play, but I like the journey they take me on—sharp, wild and stormy to restorative, calm and beautiful melodies.

I am not an instrumentalist by any means (for those who may take my words literally and think that I am one or wish to be) but I definitely am learning how to play them (poetically) to my veins for the ink in my heart to find the surface of the sun.

Whenever there was a get-together at a house, I would gravitate towards pianos. Or if someone was playing an instrument, singing or there was a cozy spot away from the crowd, that's exactly where I would be. Over the years I've come to recognize that I carry an orchestra in my soul. It is how I grasp the sentimentality, the cognitive, and emotional capacity to breathe in the life I was given and to use each instrument to unlock a window for the light to enter and unravel a new level of ink.

Music is a language I am well acquainted with for it does not need words to respond to the stories that find me in the waves. Music is pure sound with meaning like the way a baby cries at its first breath, the way whales sing in harmony, the way the leaves rustle underfoot to signal an approach, the way hope whistles from the mouth of the birds incoming, the way laughter and tears catch my attention and the way you can read me anything, show me anything, tell me anything here... when the music is on.

Gratitude as always goes to my team at *Ink Gladiators Press—Leonie Belle Hawk, Justin Adam Wolf,* and *Aelius Arche*—for always being ready to take over the tasks of layout, design, formatting, editing and proofing for me.

May the quill of hope find you in the dark,

Reena Doss

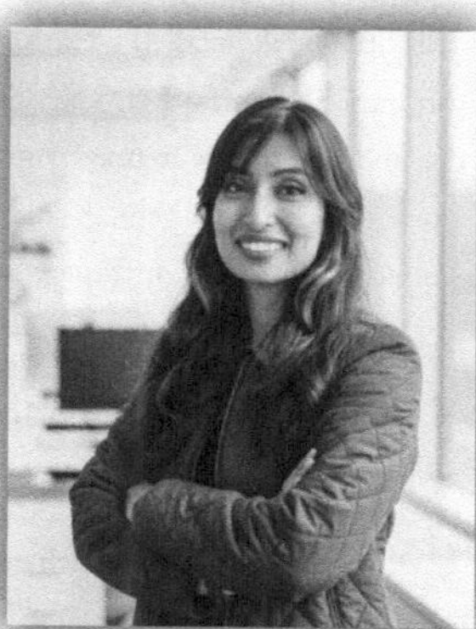

I'll find you in the dark...

Born in Calcutta with roots drawn from Chennai and Pondicherry, Reena Doss has lived most of her life in the south of India—Bangalore. Though she prefers traveling to far-off places inside her head, she sometimes ventures into the world that others call real.

Reena Doss considers writing to be her first voice of expression, followed closely by art, and creativity. Through the encouraging platform provided by the Instagram community, she reclaimed her lost voices, evolved a few others and discovered new ones along the way.

This has redeemed her trust that consistent Hope, Faith and Love in what is true ignites what is impossible to occur. Her adoration for her beloved Weaver, the Celestial Sky, Nature and her fellow Earthians has given her immeasurable courage to endure every season with a resilience born from battles overcome.

You can try and catch her but it may not always be possible as she is generally off on adventures flying on phoenix wings, swimming into the deep with mermaids and chasing fiery dragons down for stories.

To those who remain true to themselves,
to those who create magic wherever they go,
and for those who sit beside the hurt
when everyone else leaves,
Art will always immortalize you.

Please scan the QR code to follow her on Instagram @reenadossauthor
www.reenadoss.com

This little book is called a *Lantern* because love is light in disguise. It can only be found when you are buried in the dark, when the seeds die, and you choose to bravely grow and become worthy of your given name—a polished gem, a diamond that cannot help but shine. Lanterns are meant for those who need hope while they are being:

- ♥ Condemned unjustly by those who see a version they want
- ♥ Gossiped about when they are not present to defend themselves
- ♥ Taken advantage of when they were beaten down by life, by those who should have stood by them
- ♥ Judged, neglected, and persecuted while they are struggling
- ♥ Abandoned by those who willingly chose to see them as toxic because it suited their narrative
- ♥ Manipulated by those who bore false witness against them to take what wasn't theirs
- ♥ Gaslit, broken, and their truth erased while they were at their most vulnerable
- ♥ Hated, harassed, and purposefully pressured into giving up on who they are because of others' jealousy
- ♥ Trying to process trauma to speak in a language that isn't being heard
- ♥ Eagerly isolated by loved ones on the advice of others who can't understand them any more
- ♥ Neglected by those whose promises dimmed when things got difficult
- ♥ Treated as outcasts by those who expect their will to be done
- ♥ Mocked for what they do just because it is different and does not fit into any box

Promoting hope and unwrapping the stigma of mental health

For any inquiries, please email us at contact@inkgladiatorspress.com.

Please scan the QR Code below if you would like to follow us on Instagram @inkgladiatorspress.

Ink Gladiators Press®

Publishing and promoting warriors on life's battlefield

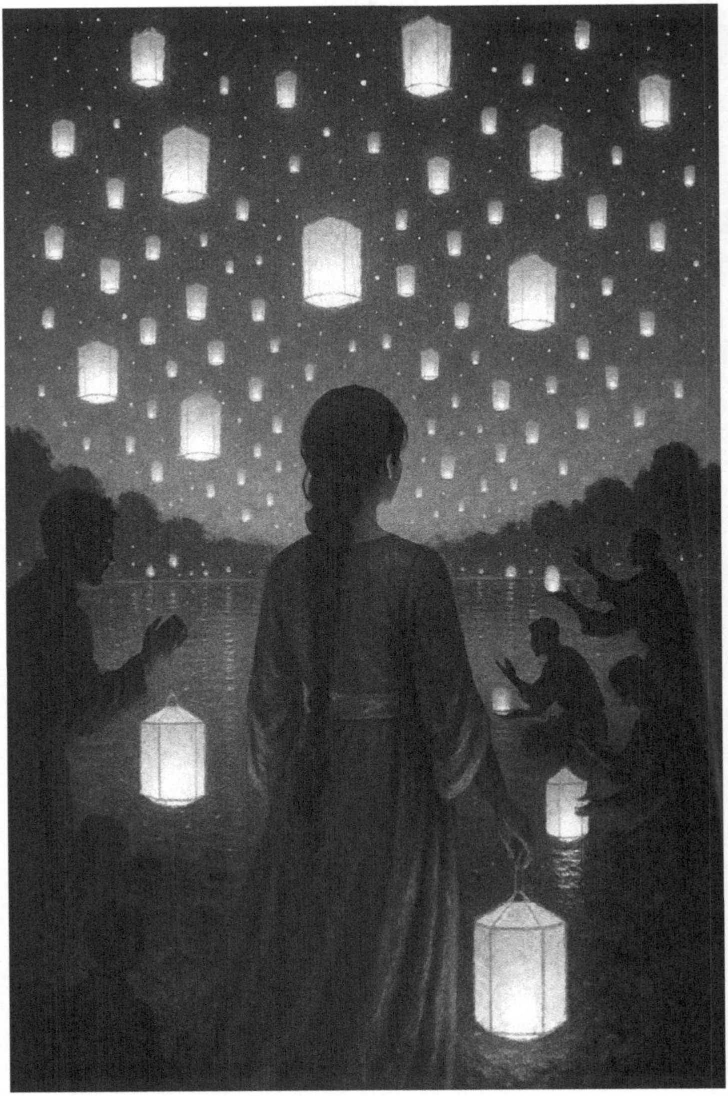

Printed at Repro India Ltd.